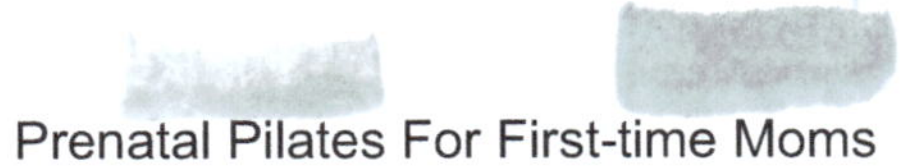

Prenatal

Pilates

For

First-time

Moms

A Transforming and Convenient pregnancy Exercise to Boost well-being and Developing Strength While at Home Using Advanced Pregnancy Pilates

Robert H. McCarthy

Table Of Contents

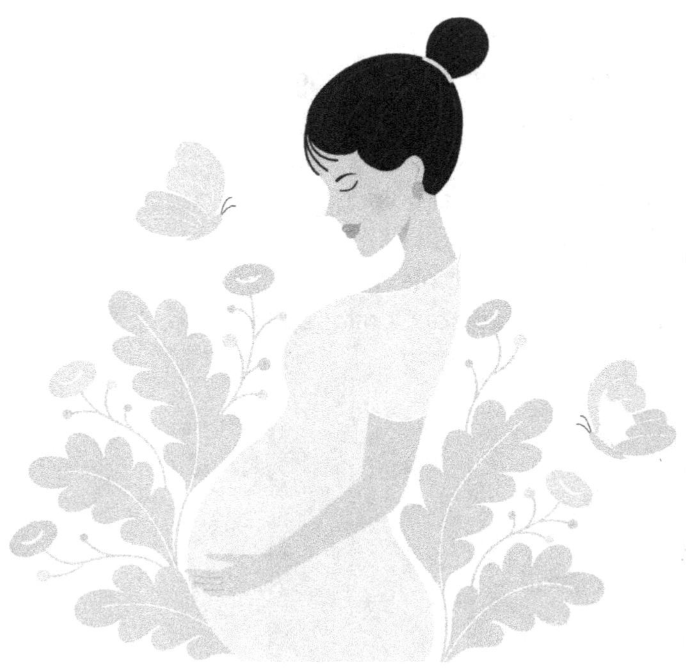

INTRODUCTION

Embracing Prenatal Pilates

Congratulations, mama-to-be, on beginning this wonderful adventure of pregnancy! As you prepare to welcome your child into the world, it's critical to consider your own health and well-being. Prenatal Pilates is a comprehensive approach to exercise during pregnancy that focuses on strengthening your body, relaxing your mind, and connecting with your growing baby.

Why Prenatal Pilates?

You may be wondering why Pilates is designed for pregnancy. The beauty of Pilates resides in its versatility and emphasis on core strength, stability, and flexibility—all of which are essential throughout pregnancy and labor. Prenatal Pilates is not only safe, but also extremely beneficial to pregnant moms, regardless of fitness level or previous workout experience.

Safe and Effective Exercise

Prenatal Pilates is a safe and effective approach to keep active throughout the three trimesters. Low-impact motions and mindful breathing methods can help relieve common discomforts like back pain, improve posture, and prepare your body for the physical demands of labor and delivery.

Building a Strong Foundation

For first-time mothers, the idea of pregnancy and childbirth may be both exhilarating and daunting. Prenatal Pilates provides a solid foundation for your parenthood journey, allowing you to embrace the changes in your body with grace and confidence. Through focused exercises and gentle stretches, you'll develop strength, resilience, and a stronger connection to your body's intrinsic intelligence.

Your Personal Workout Companion

This book is intended to be your personal companion during your prenatal Pilates adventure. Whether you're new to Pilates or an experienced practitioner, you'll discover important insights, practical ideas, and professional advice to help you every step of the way. This book will help you comprehend the basic concepts of Pilates, master crucial exercises, and navigate the specific obstacles of pregnancy.

Consultation With Your Healthcare Provider

Before beginning any workout regimen during pregnancy, you should contact your healthcare professional. Every pregnancy is unique, and your doctor or midwife can provide specific recommendations based on your medical history and current condition. Together, you can develop a safe and effective workout program that meets your requirements and interests.

Setting Realistic Goals.

As you begin your pregnant Pilates adventure, it is critical to set realistic objectives and expectations for yourself. Pregnancy is a period of great physical and mental development, and it is OK to modify your training regimen as needed to accommodate your growing body. Listen to your body's signs, accept your limitations, and enjoy each accomplishment along the road.

Creating Sacred Space

Your prenatal Pilates practice is more than simply a physical exercise; it's an opportunity to become closer to yourself and your growing baby. Find a quiet, serene area where you may disconnect from the stresses of daily life and focus on the rhythms of your body and breath. Set apart a sacred location in your house or outside where you can totally immerse yourself in the present moment.

Welcome Message:

Dear mama-to-be, welcome to your journey of loving prenatal Pilates! As you begin on this transforming journey, remember that you are not alone. This handbook is here to help you every step of the way, with insightful insights, practical ideas, and professional advice to help you manage the pleasures and challenges of pregnancy with ease and confidence. Let us begin on this lovely path of self-discovery and empowerment.

Importance of Prenatal Pilates

Prenatal Pilates is more than just another workout program; it is a comprehensive approach to fitness that is tailored to the special demands of pregnant women. Your body changes dramatically throughout pregnancy, both physically and mentally. Prenatal Pilates has several advantages that can improve your general health and prepare you for the changing experience of childbirth.

Strengthens core muscles.

The core muscles, which include the abdominals, back, and pelvic floor, are essential for supporting your developing belly and maintaining appropriate posture when pregnant. Prenatal Pilates focuses on strengthening these muscles with regulated motions and specific workouts, which can help to relieve back pain, enhance stability, and prevent common pregnancy-related symptoms.

Enhances posture and alignment.

As your body adjusts to the changes of pregnancy, you may notice changes in your posture and alignment. Prenatal Pilates focuses on perfect alignment and body awareness, allowing you to maintain ideal posture during each trimester. Strengthening the muscles that support your spine and pelvis helps lower the likelihood of postural imbalances and promote better alignment, resulting in a more pleasant pregnancy.

Improves flexibility and range of motion.

Pregnancy hormones like relaxin can increase joint laxity and cause muscular stiffness or tightness. Prenatal Pilates includes moderate stretching movements that target thigh regions including the hips, lower back, and shoulders, increasing flexibility and range of motion. Increased flexibility can improve mobility, reduce pain, and prepare your body for the physical challenges of labor and delivery.

Promotes the Mind-Body Connection

Prenatal Pilates emphasizes attentive movement and breath awareness, allowing you to connect profoundly with your body and your developing baby. Tuning into your breath and focusing on the present moment can help you feel peaceful and relaxed, minimizing the tension and worry that comes with pregnancy. This mind-body link can improve your general well-being and develop a stronger attachment with your baby.

Prepares for labor and delivery.

Prenatal Pilates skills can be useful throughout labor and delivery. Controlled breathing, visualization, and relaxation methods can help you manage discomfort and save energy throughout delivery. Pilates also improves strength, endurance, and body awareness, which can help you maintain optimal stance and support throughout birthing.

By including Pilates into your prenatal practice, you may prepare to face the changes of pregnancy with confidence, grace, and a strong feeling of connection to yourself and your growing baby.

Safety precautions

When doing pregnant Pilates, safety must always come first. While this type of exercise is typically acceptable for expecting moms, there are certain measures to take to guarantee a safe and pleasurable workout for you and your baby.

Consultation with the Healthcare Provider.

Before beginning any workout regimen during pregnancy, you should contact your healthcare professional. Your doctor or midwife can provide individualized suggestions based on your medical history, present health, and unique requirements. They may advise you on the sorts of workouts that are safe and acceptable for your stage of pregnancy, as well as any necessary adaptations.

Listen to your body.

Pregnancy is a period of great change, and your body will naturally adjust to suit your developing baby. Listen to your body's indications and respect its limits. If something causes discomfort or pain, stop immediately and adapt the workout as needed. Avoid pushing yourself past your capabilities, and put your comfort and safety first.

Avoid high-impact activities.

During pregnancy, hormonal changes cause your joints and ligaments to relax, increasing your risk of injury from high-impact activities. Prenatal Pilates focuses on low-impact movements that are easy on your joints while still providing a safe and effective method to be active throughout pregnancy. Avoid workouts that include leaping, abrupt movements, or put too much strain on the pelvic floor.

Stay hydrated and cool.

Pregnancy can lead to an increase in body temperature and fluid loss through sweating, particularly during activity. Stay hydrated by consuming lots of water before, during, and after your pregnant Pilates session. Avoid exercising in hot, humid conditions, and take breaks as needed to cool down and avoid overheating.

Modify exercises as needed.

As your pregnancy continues, you may need to adapt some routines to fit your growing body. Maintain appropriate alignment by using your core muscles and avoiding postures that compress the abdomen or hinder breathing. Props like cushions, bolsters, and resistance bands can help you support your body and improve your comfort while exercising.

Pace yourself.

Pregnancy is not the time to push yourself to your limits or aim for personal bests. Pace yourself and pay attention to your body's signs for exhaustion and exertion. Take pauses as required, and don't be afraid to alter or skip activities that seem too difficult or painful. Remember that the goal is to stay active rather than overexert yourself.

Prenatal Pilates provides numerous benefits while reducing the risk of injury and discomfort.

Prioritize safety, be aware of your body's needs, and enjoy the opportunity to connect with your baby through mindful movement and breathing.

CHAPTER 1: GETTING STARTED

Starting your prenatal Pilates adventure is an exciting and inspiring step toward a healthier, more vibrant pregnancy. Before beginning your exercises, it's critical to establish a firm foundation by learning the important concepts and concerns for practicing Pilates during pregnancy.

Planning for Your Prenatal Pilates Journey

Preparing for pregnancy Pilates entails more than simply setting up your exercise area. Take some time to consider your aims for doing Pilates while pregnant. Consider how you expect to gain from this type of exercise and what goals you want to reach. Clarifying your aims can help you stay focused and motivated during your prenatal Pilates experience.

Consultation with Healthcare Provider

Before beginning any fitness regimen while pregnant, talk with your healthcare physician. Your doctor or midwife can offer individualized advice based on your medical history, current health state, and any special pregnancy needs. Make careful to bring up any pre-existing medical issues, past pregnancy difficulties, or worries you may have about exercising while pregnant.

Setting realistic goals.

As a first-time mother, it's normal to be excited to begin your prenatal Pilates session. However, it is critical to create achievable objectives and expectations for oneself. Pregnancy is a period of tremendous change, both physically and mentally, and it is OK to modify your training regimen as needed to meet your changing demands. Kindly start with realistic objectives and progressively increase the duration and intensity of your workouts as your pregnancy advances.

Creating A Supportive Environment

Creating a supportive setting for your pregnant Pilates practice is critical to maintaining consistency and motivation. Create a designated room in your house where you can practice Pilates without distractions. Invest in a good Pilates mat and any essential props or equipment to improve your training. Consider enlisting the aid of a spouse, friend, or prenatal Pilates teacher to keep you accountable and motivated throughout the process.

Developing Your Mind-Body Connection

Prenatal Pilates is more than simply physical exercise; it also provides a chance to strengthen your mind-body connection and bond with your growing baby. Before each workout, take some time to center yourself and focus on your breathing and body. Deep breathing, visualization, and body scanning are all mindfulness exercises that may help you build a sense of calm and present.

If you are benefiting from this book you can also get the paperback version which has a specific prenatal journal just for you.

CHAPTER 2: ESSENTIAL EQUIPMENT

When it comes to pregnant Pilates, having the correct equipment may significantly improve the efficacy and comfort of your workouts. While you don't need much expensive equipment to get started, there are a few basic pieces of equipment that may help you enjoy your prenatal Pilates experience and assist your growing body throughout your pregnancy.

Pilates mat

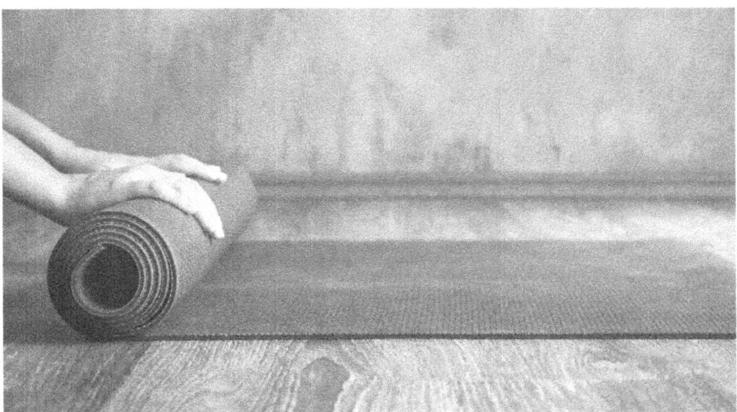

A high-quality Pilates mat serves as the foundation for your prenatal Pilates practice. Look for a mat with enough padding and support to protect your joints while also providing a comfortable surface for workouts. Choose a non-slip mat with a firm grip to avoid slipping or sliding, especially when your body changes and your center of gravity alters during pregnancy.

Supportive Props.

In addition to a Pilates mat, supporting props may improve your pregnant Pilates sessions by providing extra comfort and stability. Some crucial props to consider are:

- **Pillows**: When performing back or side workouts, use pillows to support your head, neck, and lower back. Place cushions behind your hips or between your knees to relieve discomfort and preserve appropriate alignment.

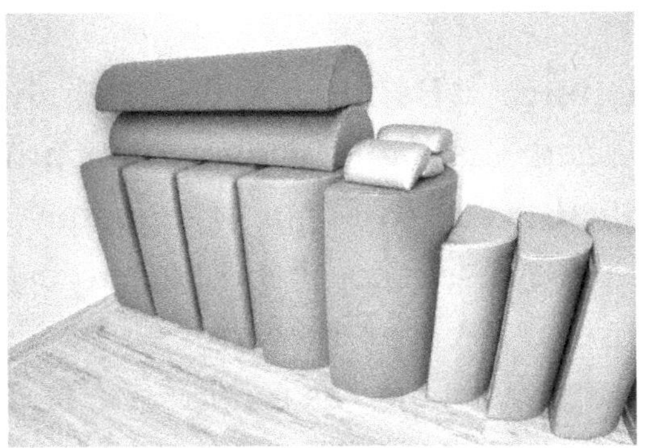

- **Bolsters**: Bolsters are adaptable props that may be used to support different portions of the body when performing exercises like sitting stretches, reclining postures, or restorative poses. Choose a bolster that provides solid support and follows your body's natural curves.

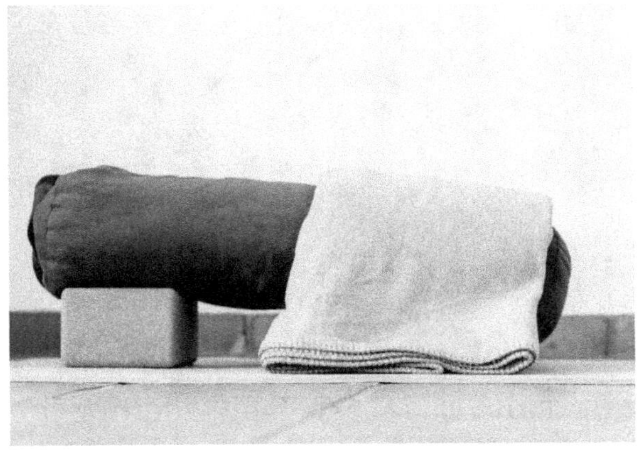

- **Resistance Bands**: These lightweight, portable, and adaptable gadgets can provide an added challenge to your pregnancy Pilates sessions. Use resistance bands to target specific muscle areas, such as the arms, legs, or glutes, and alter the resistance as required to match your strength and fitness level.

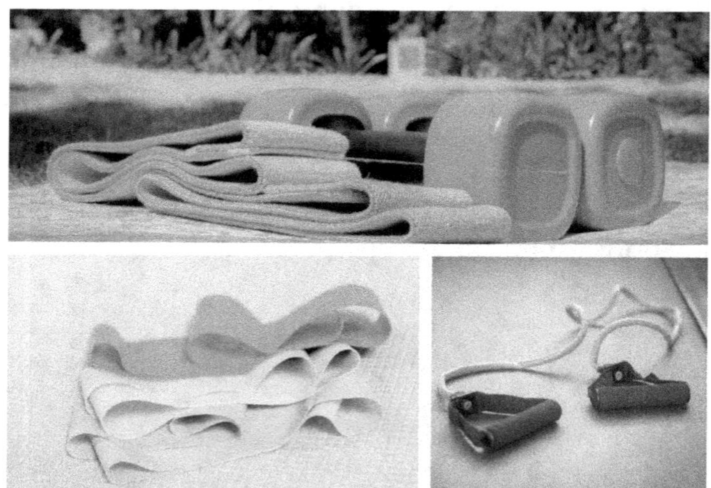

Stability Ball

A stability ball, often known as an exercise ball or Swiss ball, is an excellent addition to your pregnant Pilates toolset. Use a stability ball to conduct workouts that improve core strength, balance, and stability. Sitting on a stability ball can also help relieve lower back pain and promote good posture by exercising the core muscles.

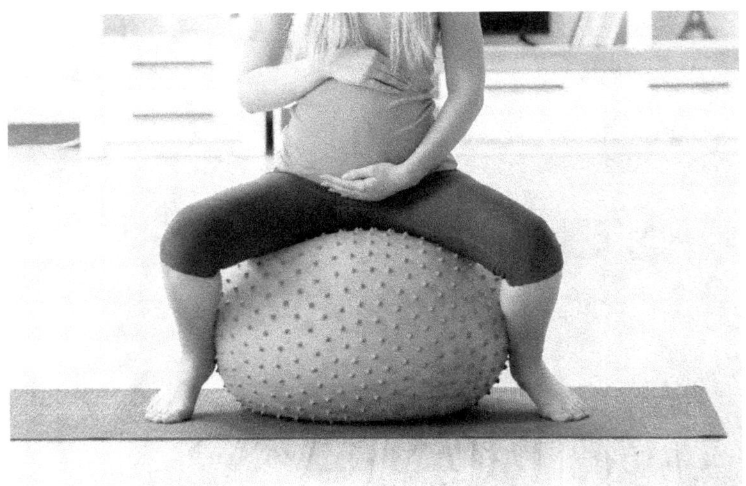

Maternity Support Belt.

As your pregnancy advances and your belly grows, you may want to consider investing in a maternity support belt. A maternal support belt gently compresses and supports the lower back and abdomen, reducing pain and improving posture during activity. Choose a maternity support belt that is adjustable, breathable, and intended to fit your growing body throughout pregnancy.

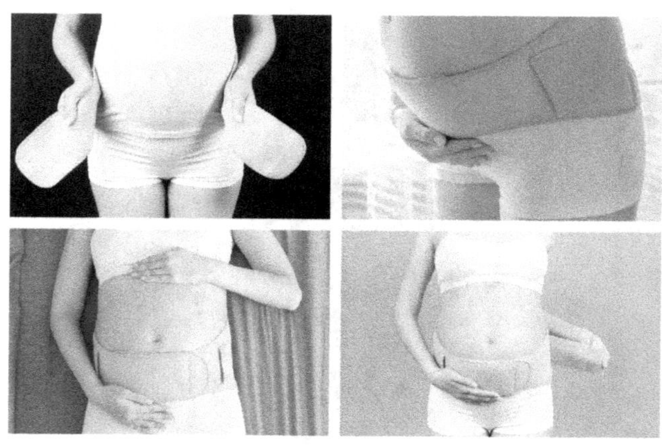

Water bottle and towel.

Staying hydrated is critical throughout pregnancy, especially when participating in vigorous activities like prenatal Pilates. To stay hydrated and maintain ideal energy levels, keep a water bottle close during your workouts and consume it on a frequent basis. Also, keep a towel ready to wipe away perspiration and be comfortable during your workout.

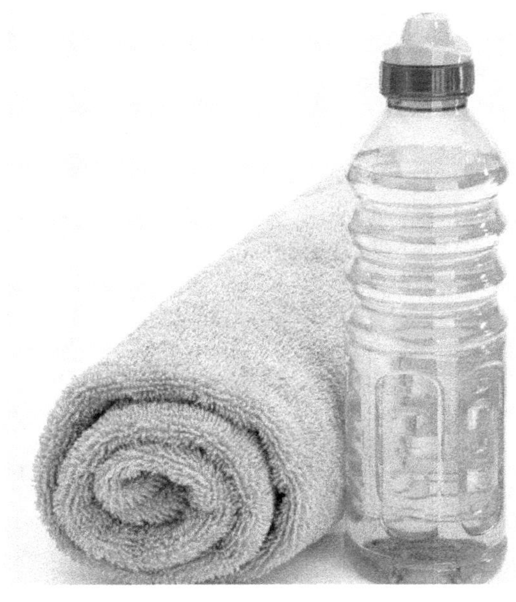

Remember to listen to your body, respect your limits, and modify your exercises as required to meet your changing demands during your pregnancy. With the correct equipment and a dedication to self-care, you may reap the myriad advantages of prenatal Pilates while also promoting a healthier, more vibrant pregnancy.

CHAPTER 3: BASIC PILATES PRINCIPLES

Pilates is founded on a set of fundamental principles that underpin all exercises and movements. Understanding and using these concepts is critical for attaining the best outcomes and maintaining a safe and productive pregnant Pilates practice. Let's look at the main Pilates concepts and how they relate to pregnancy:

Breathing Techniques.

Proper breathing is at the heart of Pilates practice, offering support, control, and relaxation with each action. Prenatal Pilates emphasizes deep diaphragmatic breathing, also known as lateral thoracic breathing. This entails breathing deeply through the nose, stretching the ribcage laterally, and expelling completely through the mouth, pulling the navel towards the spine. Conscious breathing allows oxygen to pass through the body, make you free from stress, and promotes a sense of focus and serenity, which is especially useful during pregnancy.

Core Engagement.

The core muscles, which include the abdominals, back, and pelvic floor, serve as the body's powerhouse, providing stability and support during all motions. Prenatal Pilates focuses on modest but powerful core activation to protect the spine, support the pelvis, and maintain optimal posture. Practice pulling the navel towards the spine, activating the deep transverse abdominis muscles, and elevating the pelvic floor muscles without grasping or retaining tension.

Alignment and posture.

Proper posture and alignment are critical for avoiding injury, improving general health and increasing movement efficiency. Your body's alignment changes significantly throughout pregnancy as a result of the shifting center of gravity and enlarging uterus. Maintain neutral spine posture while preserving the natural curvature of the spine, and prevent excessive arching or rounding of the back. Engage the upper back and shoulder muscles to maintain appropriate posture and decrease tension on the lower back.

Concentration and mindfulness.

Pilates is more than just going through the motions; it is about developing a profound feeling of focus and awareness with each exercise. Stay present and sensitive to your body's feelings, breath quality, and movement alignment during pregnant Pilates. By bringing awareness to your body and breath, you may strengthen proprioception, improve movement efficiency, and lessen the chance of injury.

Control and Precision.

Pilates workouts are distinguished by their accuracy and control, emphasizing the quality of movement over quantity. Prenatal Pilates emphasizes controlled, flowing movements that flow easily from one exercise to the next. Avoid abrupt or rapid motions that might strain muscles or joints, and instead concentrate on maintaining stability and control during each repeat.

Fluidity & Flow

Pilates is sometimes defined as a fluid, dynamic type of exercise that stresses seamless transitions and sustained movement. In prenatal Pilates, embrace the notion of fluidity and flow, letting your breath influence the rhythm of your exercises. Concentrate on linking one movement to the next in a smooth sequence, retaining a sense of grace and ease as your body changes and adapts during pregnancy.

Remember to approach each action with awareness, prioritize quality over quantity, and pay attention to your body's cues throughout your pregnancy. With dedication and discipline, you may use Pilates' transforming potential to improve your physical and mental health during this unique period in your life.

CHAPTER 4: WARM-UP ROUTINE.

A full warm-up is required before beginning any physical exercise, including pregnant Pilates. It helps your body prepare for the forthcoming activity by increasing blood flow to your muscles and lowering the chance of damage. In this chapter, we'll look at a gentle and efficient warm-up practice designed exclusively for pregnant moms practicing prenatal Pilates.

Gentle Joint Mobilization.

Begin your warm-up routine with modest joint mobilization activities to lubricate and extend your joints' range of motion. Begin by sitting or standing erect, feet hip-width apart, spine aligned. Then, slowly rotate your shoulders forward in little circles, gradually expanding your range of motion. Repeat this action 8-10 times, then change direction and circle your shoulders backwards.

Next, slowly twist your neck from side to side, allowing your ear to fall towards your shoulder without pushing the movement. Hold each side for a few breaths until you feel a mild stretch down the side of your neck. Continue to move your upper and lower extremity joints by performing wrist circles, ankle circles, and knee circles.

Dynamic stretches.

After moving your joints, perform dynamic stretches to lengthen and engage your muscles. Begin by standing with your feet hip-width apart and arms by your sides. Inhale while raising your arms upwards and reaching tall through your fingertips. Exhale as you drop your arms and bend forward at the hips, allowing your spine to stretch and your head to hang low.

Continue with dynamic stretches like modest side bends, hip circles, and leg swings to target your body's key muscle groups. Move slowly and thoughtfully through each stretch, keeping appropriate posture and breathing deeply into it. Repeat each dynamic stretch 8-10 times, or until you feel warmed up and ready for your pregnant Pilates session.

Mindful Breathing Awareness.

From start to end of your warm-up routine, use mindful breathing to connect with your body and relax your mind. Take slow, deep breaths in through your nose, letting your belly expand completely with each inhalation. Exhale gently through your lips, pulling your navel towards your spine to activate your core muscles. Concentrate on the sensation of your breath traveling in and out of your body, resulting in a sense of calm and presence.

As you finish your warm-up exercise, take time to assess how you're feeling physically and mentally. Take note of any tense or uncomfortable regions in your body, as well as your energy and attitude. By focusing on your body and breath, you may improve the efficiency of your pregnant Pilates session and create a good tone for the rest of your practice.

CHAPTER 5: MAIN WORKOUT

The primary workout is the core of your prenatal Pilates practice, and it consists of a sequence of movements meant to strengthen your body, increase flexibility, and improve your general well-being while pregnant. In this chapter, we'll look at fundamental Pilates exercises designed expressly for first-time mothers, as well as adjustments and variants to suit different trimesters and fitness levels.

Pelvic Floor Muscle Exercise

The Hundred is a basic Pilates exercise that strengthens the core, improves circulation, and boosts endurance. To begin the Modified Hundred while pregnant, lie on your back with your knees bent and feet flat on the mat. Engage your core muscles and lift your head, neck, and shoulders off the mat, keeping your arms straight alongside your body.

Begin pumping your arms up and down in short, controlled motions, inhaling and exhaling for five counts each. Throughout the workout, focus on core stability and deep, rhythmic breathing. To accommodate pregnancy, keep your head and shoulders supported with a pillow or cushion to relieve strain on your neck and spine.

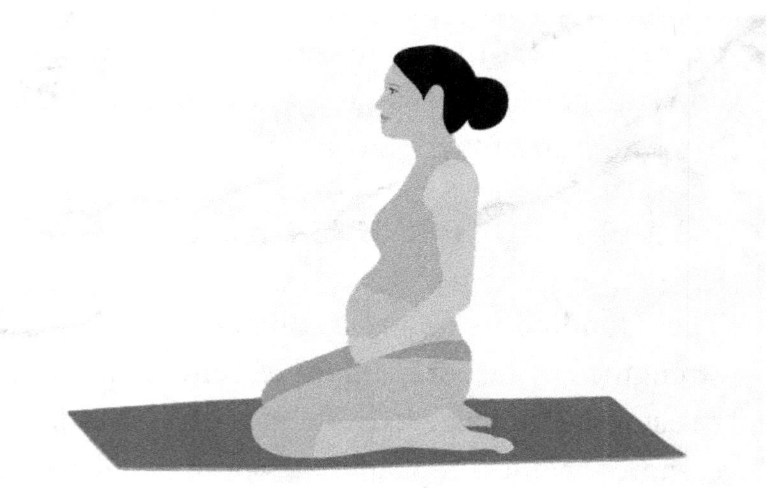

Pelvic Tilts

Pelvic tilts are a great exercise for strengthening the deep abdominal muscles and stabilizing the pelvis, which can assist with lower back discomfort and posture during pregnancy. Begin by laying on your back, legs bent, and feet flat on the mat. Inhale to prepare, then exhale while tilting your pelvis toward your belly button and flattening your lower back into the mat.

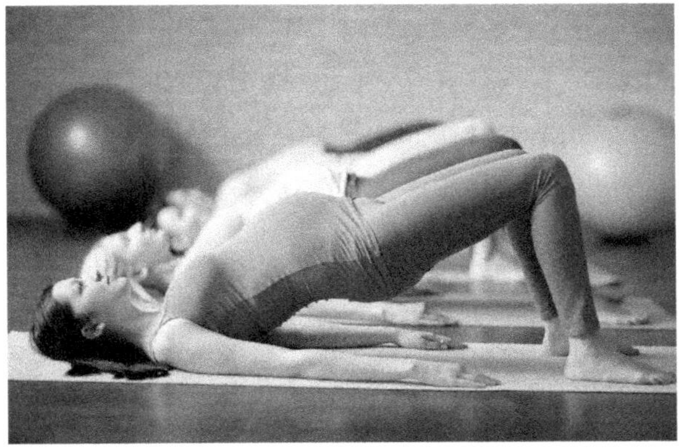

Inhale to release the tilt and return to neutral, then exhale while tilting your pelvis in the other direction and arching your lower back slightly away from the mat. Continue to go through pelvic tilts while breathing, concentrating on keeping a smooth, controlled motion and utilizing your core muscles throughout.

Cat-Cow Stretch.

The Cat-Cow Stretch is a moderate yoga-inspired exercise that relieves back strain, increases flexibility, and promotes calm during pregnancy. Begin in a tabletop posture with your wrists immediately under your shoulders and your knees beneath your hips. Inhale as you arch your back, lowering your belly to the mat and raising your head and tailbone to the ceiling (Cow Pose).

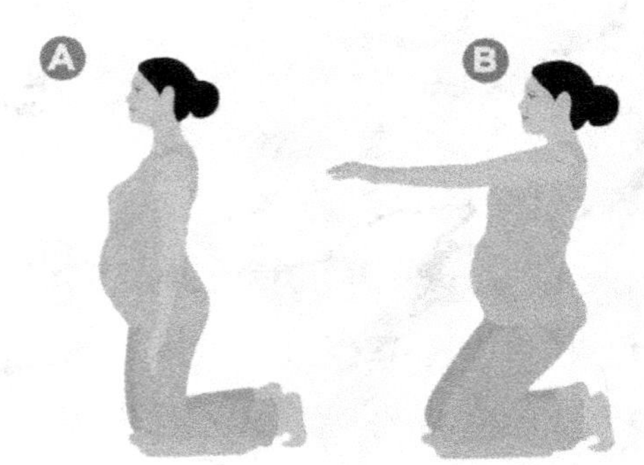

Exhale while rounding your back, tucking your chin into your chest and bringing your belly button toward your spine (Cat Pose). Move through the Cat-Cow Stretch with your breath, effortlessly transitioning between the two postures and focusing on generating room and mobility in your spine.

Upper Back Stretch

Improves your posture.

Sit cross-legged, back upright, and hands behind your head.

Inhale gently.

As you exhale, draw in your belly and stretch your back while looking up at the ceiling. Take another breath by compressing your shoulders and return to the beginning posture.

Repeat five to 10 times.

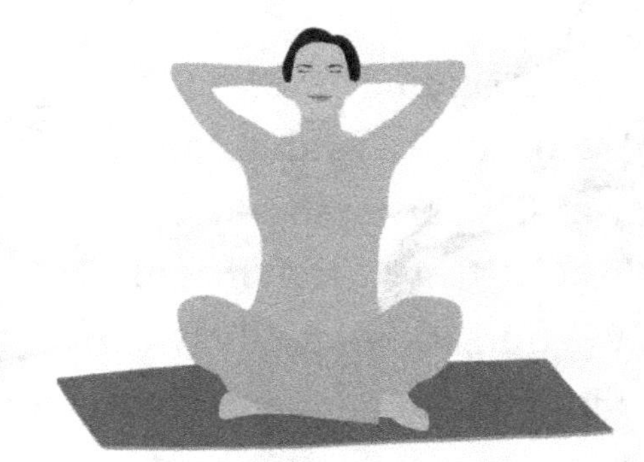

Thigh Stretch

Strengthens the abdominal muscles, lower back, hips, and buttocks.

Kneel down on a carpet or mat, hip-width apart, and draw in your abs. Lean back, breathe in, and pinch your buttocks. Raise your arms parallel to the floor, palms facing down. Breathe out as you drop your arms down.

Return to the starting position.

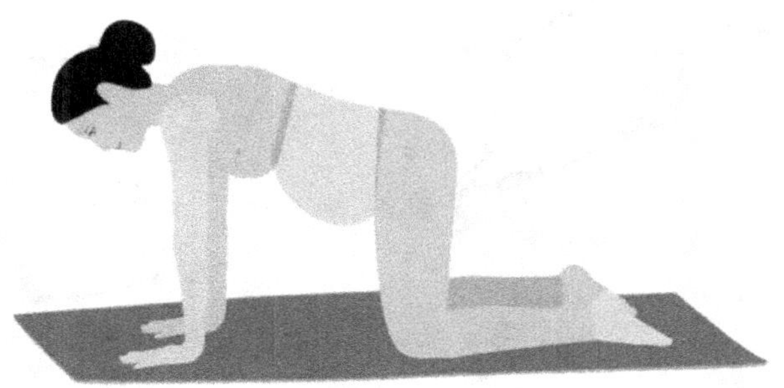

The Sword

Improves balance and strengthens the abdominals, back, and legs. Stand with your feet apart and broader than your hips.

Bend your knees and transfer your right hand to the left knee, as illustrated in the image.

Now raise your right hand upwards to the right, as if you were removing a sword from your hip belt. Continue to glance at the hand while doing so. Repeat with your left side.

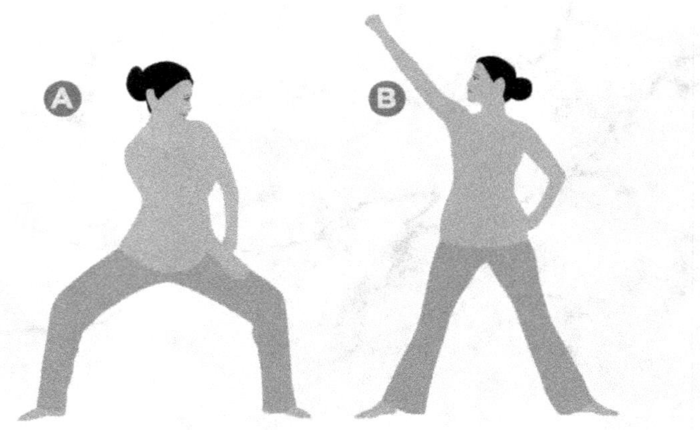

Sword Arm

Improves balance and strengthens the abdominals, arms, back, and hips.

Kneel with your right knee and both hands on the floor. Stretch the left leg with the abs pushed in and the hips looking upward.

Inhale as you draw your left hand to the sky and glance up at your hand.

Exhale by lowering your hand back to its original position.

Switch to the left side and repeat.

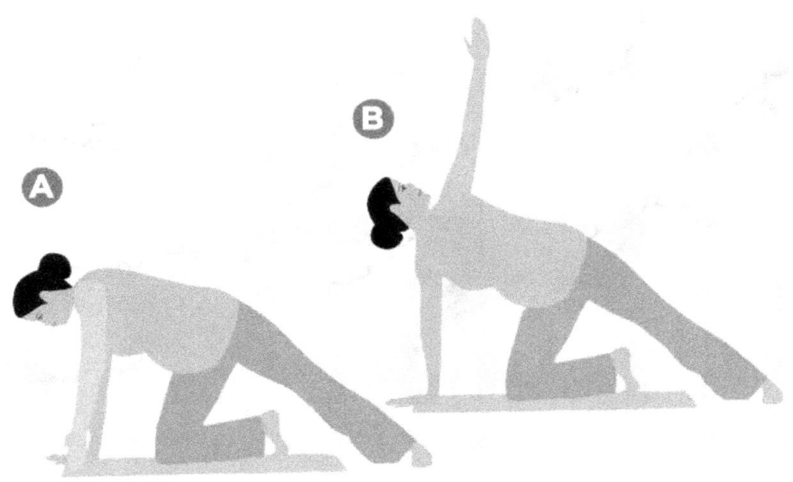

Wagging The Tail

Increases flexibility and stability while strengthening the lower back and abdominals.

Begin on all fours, keeping your wrists aligned with the shoulders. Suck in your tummy, raise one knee, and do circular movements with the leg.

Repeat with the opposite leg. Repeat three to four times.

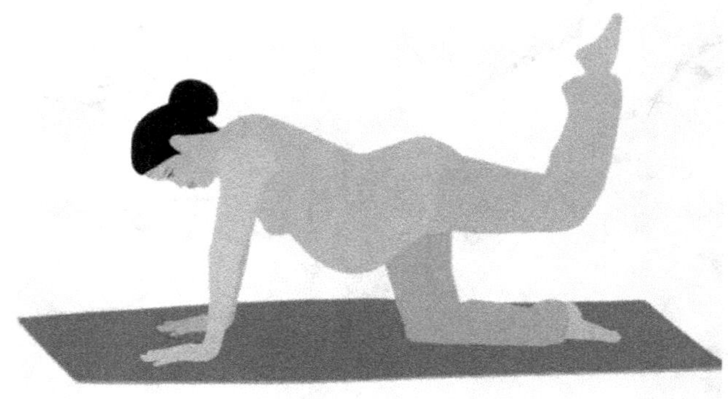

Deep Tummy Strengthening

Increases back support.

Lie on one side with the knees slightly bent. Breathe in and breathe out. And try to pull in the tummy towards the spine.

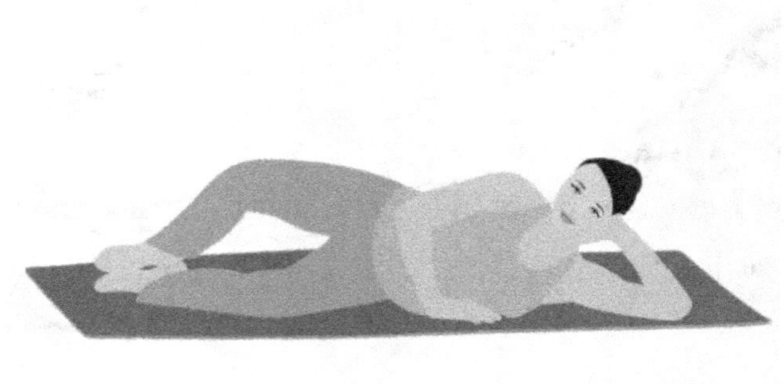

Modifications and variations

Throughout your prenatal Pilates practice, you must listen to your body and change workouts as needed to meet your changing demands and comfort level. As your pregnancy continues, you may need to modify the intensity, duration, and range of motion of specific activities. Below are some general adjustments and alterations to consider:

- **Use Props**: Use cushions, bolsters, and resistance bands to give support, stability, and additional resistance during workouts.
- **Adjust Range of Motion**: Reduce the range of motion or intensity of workouts as necessary to avoid strain or pain, especially as your pregnancy advances.
- **Experiment** with several postures, such as standing, sitting, or hands and knees, to see which is most comfortable and beneficial for your body.
- **Concentrate on Alignment**: Pay special attention to your alignment and posture

throughout each exercise, and avoid postures that place too much strain on your joints or jeopardize your stability.

By including these fundamental Pilates movements into your prenatal workouts and making necessary adaptations, you may strengthen your body, increase flexibility, and improve general well-being throughout pregnancy. Remember to be attentive, listen to your body, and enjoy the experience of nourishing yourself and your growing baby with prenatal Pilates.

CHAPTER 6: COOL DOWN AND STRETCHING

After you've finished your primary pregnant Pilates practice, be sure to cool down and stretch properly. Cooling down allows your heart rate and respiration to gradually return to normal, whilst stretching relieves muscular tension, increases flexibility, and promotes relaxation. In this chapter, we'll examine a gentle and efficient cool down and stretching program created exclusively for pregnant women.

Seated Spinal Twist.

Begin your cool down and stretching exercise in a comfortable sitting position on the mat. Sit tall, legs out in front of you, spine elongated. Inhale to stretch your spine, then exhale and slowly rotate to the right, with your left hand on your right knee and your right hand behind you for support.

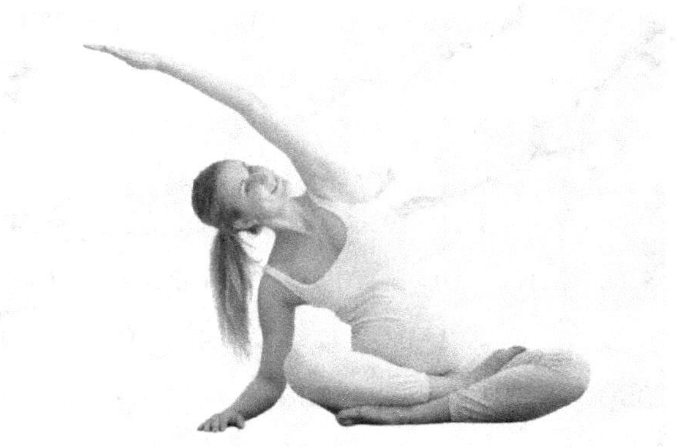

Hold the twist for a few breaths to feel a nice stretch along the sides of your body and spine. Inhale to return to center, then exhale as you rotate to the left, with your right hand on your knee and your left hand behind you. Hold the twist for a few breaths before returning to center. Repeat the sitting spinal twist on both sides, moving gently and deliberately while you breathe.

Child's Pose

From a sitting posture, go into Child's Pose to stretch and relieve tension in your lower back, hips, and shoulders. Kneel on your mat, keeping your knees hip-width apart and your toes together, then sit back on your heels. Inhale to lengthen your spine, then exhale as you fold forward, dropping your chest between your thighs and stretching your arms out in front of you.

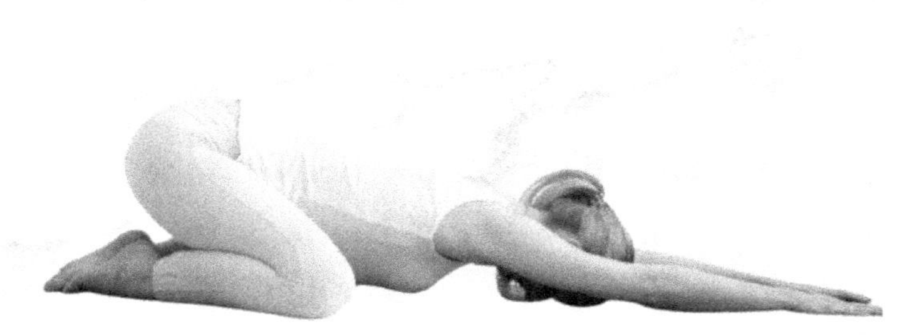

Rest your forehead on the mat and let your chest descend to the ground, experiencing a gentle stretch down your spine and hips. Take calm, deep breaths while holding the posture for 30 seconds to 1 minute, allowing your body to relax and release tension with each exhale.

Cat-Cow Stretch.

Return to a tabletop posture on your hands and knees, then perform a few rounds of Cat-Cow Stretch to relieve tension in your spine and enhance mobility. Inhale as you arch your back, lowering your belly to the mat and raising your head and tailbone to the ceiling (Cow Pose). Exhale while rounding your back, tucking your chin into your chest and bringing your belly button toward your spine (Cat Pose).

Move gently and gracefully between the Cat and Cow poses, keeping your motions in tune with your breath. With each inhale, focus on generating space and length in your spine, while exhaling releases tension and rigidity.

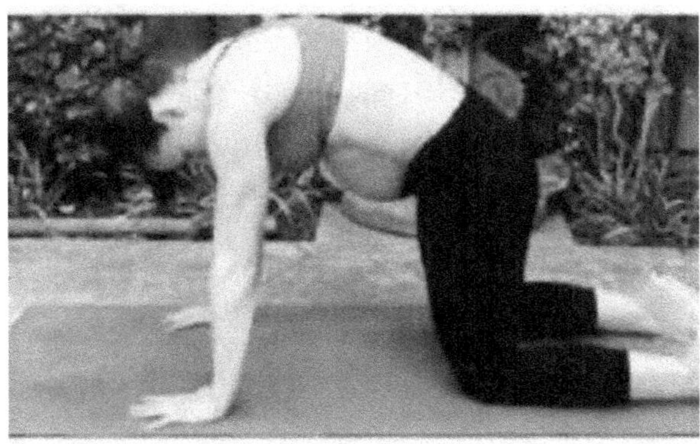

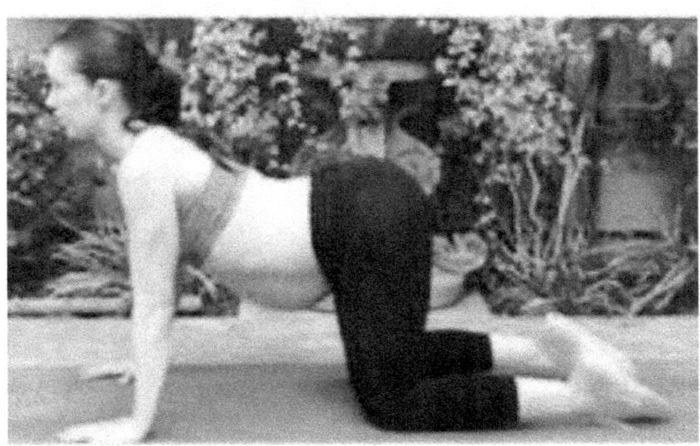

Supported forward fold.

From the tabletop position, take a sit position on your mat with your legs stretched in front of you. Sit tall with your spine extended, then inhale to lengthen it even more. Exhale as you tilt forward at the hips, folding your torso over your legs and extending your hands to your feet.

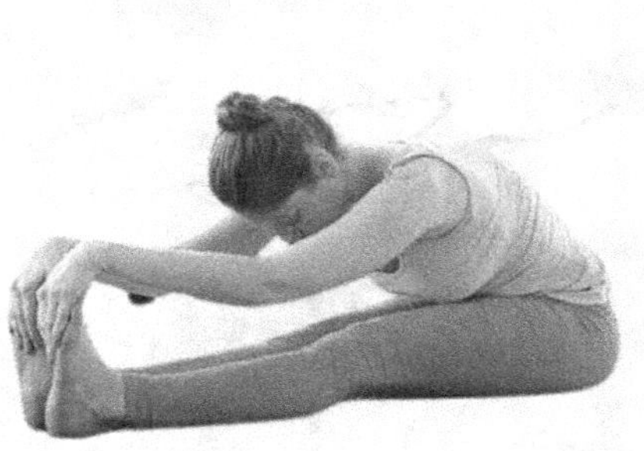

If necessary, use cushions or bolsters to support your body and head during the forward fold, allowing you to fully relax into the stretch. Hold the forward fold for 30 seconds to a minute, inhaling deeply and letting your body release tension with each exhalation.

Hip Opener Stretch

Finish your cool-down and stretching regimen with a moderate hip opening stretch to relieve tension in your hips and pelvis. Lie on your back, knees bent and feet flat on the mat, then cross your right ankle over your left knee in a figure-four posture.

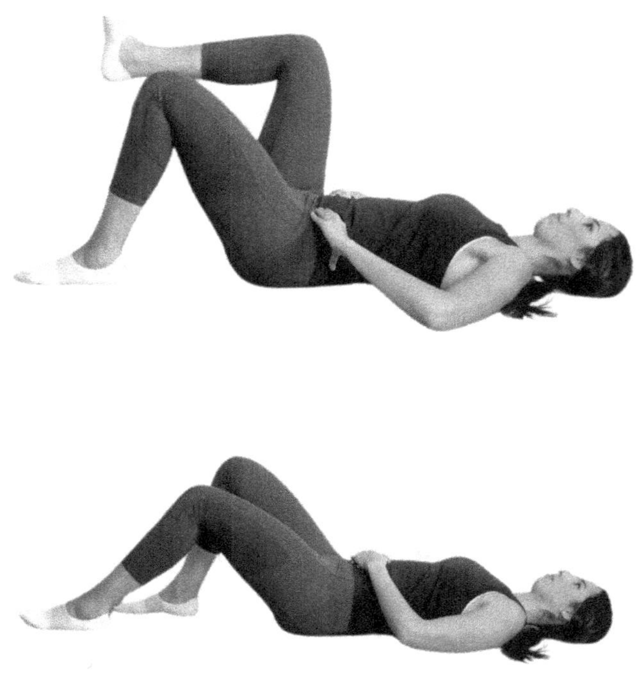

Thread your right hand through the gap between your legs, then interlace your fingers behind your left thigh while gently pushing your left knee towards your chest. Keep your right knee extended to the side to increase the stretch in your right hip. Hold the stretch for 30 seconds to 1 minute before switching sides and repeating on the opposite side.

Modifications and variations

Throughout your cool down and stretching regimen, listen to your body and make alterations as required to maintain comfort and safety. Below are some general adjustments and alterations to consider:

- **Use Props**: Pillows, bolsters, or yoga blocks can help you stretch while also providing comfort and stability.
- **Modify Intensity**: Vary the intensity and length of stretches according to your comfort level and flexibility, especially as your pregnancy advances.

- **Concentrate on Breath**: Throughout your cool down and stretching procedure, breathe deeply and mindfully to relax and release tension.

Remember to walk carefully, breathe deeply, and pay attention to your body's cues while you stretch and relax to nourish yourself and your developing baby.

CHAPTER 7: THE MIND-BODY CONNECTION

The mind-body link is central to Pilates practice, emphasizing the need of developing awareness, focus, and purpose in all movements. In this chapter, we'll look at how the mind-body connection affects prenatal Pilates and how you may use it to improve your physical and mental health throughout pregnancy.

Promoting Awareness

Prenatal Pilates offers a unique chance to increase your knowledge of your body and its requirements while pregnant. Mindful movement and breath awareness allow you to tune into the subtle feelings, rhythms, and changes in your body, building a stronger connection and knowledge of yourself and your growing baby. Cultivating awareness helps you to move more precisely, controllably, and efficiently, while also lowering your chance of injury and boosting overall exercise safety.

Fostering Mindfulness

Mindfulness is the discipline of being totally present in the moment, without judgment or distraction, and is central to Pilates philosophy. Mindfulness in prenatal Pilates enables you to approach each exercise with curiosity, openness, and acceptance, helping you to completely connect with your body and breath. Practicing mindfulness can help you reduce stress and anxiety, increase attention and focus, and cultivate a sense of peace and well-being during your pregnancy.

Setting Intention.

Setting intentions is an effective way to guide your pregnant Pilates practice and link your actions with your beliefs and goals. Before commencing each activity, take time to consider your goals for the session—whether they are to improve your body, relieve discomfort, or just bond with your baby. Setting specific objectives allows you to concentrate your energy and attention, stay motivated and inspired, and get more meaning and fulfillment out of your practice.

Listen to Your Body

Your body is continuously providing you signs and cues about its demands and limits, and learning to listen to them is critical for practicing pregnant Pilates safely and successfully. Pay close attention to how your body feels throughout each action and respond to its input by making modifications as needed to suit your comfort and energy level. Listening to your body with love and respect allows you to avoid overexertion, injury, and promotes a happy and loving experience for both you and your baby.

Embracing The Connection

The mind-body connection in prenatal Pilates goes beyond the physical to include the emotional and spiritual aspects of pregnancy. Accept the connection between your mind, body, and spirit as you perform each exercise, allowing you to tap into a stronger sense of purpose, strength, and resilience. By acknowledging the link between your mind and body, you may develop a stronger feeling of self-awareness, empowerment, and faith in your body's intrinsic wisdom to lead you through the magical adventure of pregnancy and labor.

Incorporating the mind-body connection into your prenatal Pilates practice may enhance your experience, strengthen your bond with yourself and your baby, and prepare you to face the transforming adventure of pregnancy with grace and confidence.

CHAPTER 8: POSTNATAL CONSIDERATIONS

The postnatal phase is a period of transition and adjustment in which your body heals after delivery and adjusts to the responsibilities of caring for a baby.

Gradual Return to Exercise.

Following childbirth, it is critical to approach exercise with compassion, tenderness, and respect for your body's healing process. In the early postpartum period, focus on soft, low-impact activities like walking, pelvic floor exercises, and gentle stretching. As you progressively acquire strength and endurance, you can gradually resume more difficult activities, such as postnatal Pilates, with the help of your healthcare professional.

Transition to Postnatal Pilates

As your body heals and recovers from delivery, you may want to continue your Pilates practice. To transition to postnatal Pilates, begin with easy, adjusted movements that focus on core strength, pelvic floor stability, and total body fitness. Begin with a postnatal Pilates class tailored to new mothers, or work with a qualified postnatal Pilates teacher who can offer individualized advice and support based on your unique requirements and fitness level.

Concentrate on the core and pelvic floor.

During pregnancy and childbirth, the muscles of the core and pelvic floor alter significantly, becoming weaker or strained. Postnatal Pilates can help rebuild strength, stability, and coordination in these key muscle groups, therefore promoting healing and lowering the likelihood of common postpartum disorders like diastasis recti and urine incontinence. To restore your core's balance and function, focus on activities that target the deep abdominal muscles, pelvic floor muscles, and back and hip muscles.

Recovery Tips

In addition to exercise, there are various rehabilitation strategies that can aid in your postpartum healing journey:

- Prioritize relaxation and sleep whenever possible to help your body recover and maintain its energy levels.
- Maintain hydration and nutrition with a well-balanced diet high in nutrient-dense foods to promote healing and restore lost nutrients.
- Use mild self-massage or instruments like foam rollers or massage balls to relieve tension and improve circulation in stiff or tight muscles.
- Incorporate relaxation techniques like deep breathing, meditation, or moderate yoga into your daily routine to reduce stress and improve emotional well-being.

Listen to your body.

As you restart exercise after childbirth, pay attention to your body's indications and alter your routines accordingly. Pay attention to your physical and emotional reactions before and after exercise, and respect your body's need for rest, recuperation, and food. If you suffer any pain, discomfort, or strange symptoms, discontinue exercise and communicate with your healthcare physician for proper diagnosis and assistance.

Seek professional guidance.

If you're not sure how to safely start exercising after childbirth, or if you have specific concerns or issues, see a certified healthcare professional or postnatal fitness specialist. A physical therapist, pelvic health expert, or qualified postnatal Pilates teacher can offer tailored advice, assessments, and support to help you navigate the postpartum period with confidence and ease.

Incorporating these postnatal factors into your Pilates practice can help your body recover and heal, develop strength and stability, and improve general well-being throughout the transforming postpartum time. Remember to approach exercise with patience, love, and self-compassion, and to appreciate each step forward on your path to postpartum health and vitality.

CONCLUSION

Congratulations on finishing "Prenatal Pilates for First-Time Moms"! As you conclude this chapter, consider the information obtained, the activities attempted, and the connections created between mind, body, and spirit. In this last chapter, we'll celebrate your accomplishments, recognize the transforming effect of Pilates throughout pregnancy, and provide support for the road ahead.

Recap of Key Points

Throughout this book, you've learned about the great advantages of prenatal Pilates for first-time mothers, including increased strength and flexibility, relaxation, and mindfulness. You've learned how to practice Pilates safely and successfully while pregnant, taking into account your body's particular requirements and changes as you prepare for your baby's arrival.

Key points to remember are:

- *Prenatal Pilates emphasizes optimal alignment, breathing methods, and core activation.*
- *The importance of listening to your body, making adjustments as appropriate, and emphasizing safety and comfort.*
- *The importance of awareness, intention, and connection in developing a satisfying and empowering Pilates practice.*
- *Postnatal Pilates can help with recuperation, strength growth, and overall well-being after childbirth.*

Encouragement of Continued Practice

As you begin on the next chapter of your journey—whether it's ushering your baby into the world, navigating the pleasures and challenges of parenthood, or just continuing to prioritize self-care and well-being—remember the lessons learned and habits developed through prenatal Pilates.

Remember to listen to your body, respect your limitations, and believe in your natural power and perseverance. Remember to breathe deeply, walk deliberately, and maintain awareness and presence in every moment. Remember that you are capable, supported, and deserving of love and care, both from yourself and others around you.

As you go ahead, may you take the knowledge and grace of prenatal Pilates with you, welcoming the journey with bravery, compassion, and pleasure. May you discover courage in your vulnerabilities, beauty in your flaws, and serenity in knowing that you are precisely where you are supposed to be.

Thank you for letting us be a part of your pregnancy Pilates adventure. May it continue to nourish and inspire you as you begin on the incredible journey of parenting. I wish you health, happiness, and plentiful blessings in the days and years ahead.

With love and thanks.
Robert H. McCarthy

Could you please take a moment to leave a review. Thank you

My prenatal Journal

Today's goal ______________________________   **Date:** __________

Mood/Emotion Tracker

◯ ◯ ◯ ◯ ◯

VERRY SAD ⟷ VERY HAPPY

How did you feel physically during today's prenatal Pilates session?

Did you notice any changes in your body's flexibility or strength since starting prenatal Pilates?

What thoughts or emotions arose during your prenatal Pilates session?

Space for Creativity
(DOODLES, ILLUSTRATION, TEXT,ETC)

How do you plan to integrate what you've learned in today's session into your daily routine?

How did practicing prenatal Pilates today make you feel about your pregnancy journey?

My prenatal Journal

Today's goal _________________________________ **Date:** __________

Mood/Emotion Tracker

◯ ◯ ◯ ◯ ◯

VERRY SAD ⟷ VERY HAPPY

How did you feel physically during today's prenatal Pilates session?

Did you notice any changes in your body's flexibility or strength since starting prenatal Pilates?

What thoughts or emotions arose during your prenatal Pilates session?

Space for Creativity
(DOODLES, ILLUSTRATION, TEXT,ETC)

How do you plan to integrate what you've learned in today's session into your daily routine?

How did practicing prenatal Pilates today make you feel about your pregnancy journey?

My prenatal Journal

Today's goal _______________________________   **Date:** _________

Mood/Emotion Tracker

◯ ◯ ◯ ◯ ◯

VERRY SAD ⟷ VERY HAPPY

How did you feel physically during today's prenatal Pilates session?

Did you notice any changes in your body's flexibility or strength since starting prenatal Pilates?

What thoughts or emotions arose during your prenatal Pilates session?

Space for Creativity
(DOODLES, ILLUSTRATION, TEXT,ETC)

How do you plan to integrate what you've learned in today's session into your daily routine?

How did practicing prenatal Pilates today make you feel about your pregnancy journey?

My prenatal Journal

Today's goal ___________________________________ **Date:** ___________

Mood/Emotion Tracker

◯ ◯ ◯ ◯ ◯

VERRY SAD ⟵⟶ VERY HAPPY

How did you feel physically during today's prenatal Pilates session?

Space for Creativity
(DOODLES, ILLUSTRATION, TEXT,ETC)

Did you notice any changes in your body's flexibility or strength since starting prenatal Pilates?

How do you plan to integrate what you've learned in today's session into your daily routine?

What thoughts or emotions arose during your prenatal Pilates session?

How did practicing prenatal Pilates today make you feel about your pregnancy journey?

My prenatal Journal

Today's goal _______________________________   Date: _________

Mood/Emotion Tracker

◯ ◯ ◯ ◯ ◯

VERRY SAD ⟵⟶ VERY HAPPY

How did you feel physically during today's prenatal Pilates session?

Did you notice any changes in your body's flexibility or strength since starting prenatal Pilates?

What thoughts or emotions arose during your prenatal Pilates session?

Space for Creativity
(DOODLES, ILLUSTRATION, TEXT,ETC)

How do you plan to integrate what you've learned in today's session into your daily routine?

How did practicing prenatal Pilates today make you feel about your pregnancy journey?

My prenatal Journal

Today's goal _________________________________   Date: __________

Mood/Emotion Tracker

◯ ◯ ◯ ◯ ◯

VERRY SAD ⟵⟶ VERY HAPPY

How did you feel physically during today's prenatal Pilates session?

Did you notice any changes in your body's flexibility or strength since starting prenatal Pilates?

What thoughts or emotions arose during your prenatal Pilates session?

Space for Creativity
(DOODLES, ILLUSTRATION, TEXT,ETC)

How do you plan to integrate what you've learned in today's session into your daily routine?

How did practicing prenatal Pilates today make you feel about your pregnancy journey?

My prenatal Journal

Today's goal _______________________________   **Date:** _________

Mood/Emotion Tracker

○ ○ ○ ○ ○

VERRY SAD ⟷ VERY HAPPY

How did you feel physically during today's prenatal Pilates session?

Did you notice any changes in your body's flexibility or strength since starting prenatal Pilates?

What thoughts or emotions arose during your prenatal Pilates session?

Space for Creativity
(DOODLES, ILLUSTRATION, TEXT,ETC)

How do you plan to integrate what you've learned in today's session into your daily routine?

How did practicing prenatal Pilates today make you feel about your pregnancy journey?

My prenatal Journal

Today's goal _________________________________ Date: _________

Mood/Emotion Tracker

◯ ◯ ◯ ◯ ◯

VERRY SAD ⟵⟶ VERY HAPPY

How did you feel physically during today's prenatal Pilates session?

Did you notice any changes in your body's flexibility or strength since starting prenatal Pilates?

What thoughts or emotions arose during your prenatal Pilates session?

Space for Creativity
(DOODLES, ILLUSTRATION, TEXT,ETC)

How do you plan to integrate what you've learned in today's session into your daily routine?

How did practicing prenatal Pilates today make you feel about your pregnancy journey?

My prenatal Journal

Today's goal ___________________________ **Date:** _________

Mood/Emotion Tracker

◯ ◯ ◯ ◯ ◯

VERRY SAD ⟷ VERY HAPPY

How did you feel physically during today's prenatal Pilates session?

Did you notice any changes in your body's flexibility or strength since starting prenatal Pilates?

What thoughts or emotions arose during your prenatal Pilates session?

Space for Creativity
(DOODLES, ILLUSTRATION, TEXT,ETC)

How do you plan to integrate what you've learned in today's session into your daily routine?

How did practicing prenatal Pilates today make you feel about your pregnancy journey?

My prenatal Journal

Today's goal ___________________________________   Date: ___________

Mood/Emotion Tracker

○ ○ ○ ○ ○

VERRY SAD ⟷ VERY HAPPY

How did you feel physically during today's prenatal Pilates session?

Did you notice any changes in your body's flexibility or strength since starting prenatal Pilates?

What thoughts or emotions arose during your prenatal Pilates session?

Space for Creativity
(DOODLES, ILLUSTRATION, TEXT,ETC)

How do you plan to integrate what you've learned in today's session into your daily routine?

How did practicing prenatal Pilates today make you feel about your pregnancy journey?

My prenatal Journal

Today's goal _______________________________   **Date:** _________

Mood/Emotion Tracker

○ ○ ○ ○ ○

VERRY SAD ⟷ VERY HAPPY

How did you feel physically during today's prenatal Pilates session?

Did you notice any changes in your body's flexibility or strength since starting prenatal Pilates?

What thoughts or emotions arose during your prenatal Pilates session?

Space for Creativity
(DOODLES, ILLUSTRATION, TEXT,ETC)

How do you plan to integrate what you've learned in today's session into your daily routine?

How did practicing prenatal Pilates today make you feel about your pregnancy journey?

My prenatal Journal

Today's goal ___________________________________ Date: __________

Mood/Emotion Tracker

○ ○ ○ ○ ○

VERRY SAD ⟷ VERY HAPPY

How did you feel physically during today's prenatal Pilates session?

Did you notice any changes in your body's flexibility or strength since starting prenatal Pilates?

What thoughts or emotions arose during your prenatal Pilates session?

Space for Creativity
(DOODLES, ILLUSTRATION, TEXT,ETC)

How do you plan to integrate what you've learned in today's session into your daily routine?

How did practicing prenatal Pilates today make you feel about your pregnancy journey?

My prenatal Journal

Today's goal _________________________________ Date: __________

Mood/Emotion Tracker

◯ ◯ ◯ ◯ ◯

VERRY SAD ⟷ VERY HAPPY

How did you feel physically during today's prenatal Pilates session?

Did you notice any changes in your body's flexibility or strength since starting prenatal Pilates?

What thoughts or emotions arose during your prenatal Pilates session?

Space for Creativity
(DOODLES, ILLUSTRATION, TEXT,ETC)

How do you plan to integrate what you've learned in today's session into your daily routine?

How did practicing prenatal Pilates today make you feel about your pregnancy journey?

My prenatal Journal

Today's goal _________________________________   **Date:** _________

Mood/Emotion Tracker

○ ○ ○ ○ ○

VERRY SAD ⟷ VERY HAPPY

How did you feel physically during today's prenatal Pilates session?

Did you notice any changes in your body's flexibility or strength since starting prenatal Pilates?

What thoughts or emotions arose during your prenatal Pilates session?

Space for Creativity
(DOODLES, ILLUSTRATION, TEXT,ETC)

How do you plan to integrate what you've learned in today's session into your daily routine?

How did practicing prenatal Pilates today make you feel about your pregnancy journey?

My prenatal Journal

Today's goal _______________________________ Date: _________

Mood/Emotion Tracker

◯ ◯ ◯ ◯ ◯

VERRY SAD ⟷ VERY HAPPY

How did you feel physically during today's prenatal Pilates session?

Did you notice any changes in your body's flexibility or strength since starting prenatal Pilates?

What thoughts or emotions arose during your prenatal Pilates session?

Space for Creativity
(DOODLES, ILLUSTRATION, TEXT,ETC)

How do you plan to integrate what you've learned in today's session into your daily routine?

How did practicing prenatal Pilates today make you feel about your pregnancy journey?

My prenatal Journal

Today's goal _______________________________   Date: _______

Mood/Emotion Tracker

○ ○ ○ ○ ○

VERRY SAD ←——→ VERY HAPPY

How did you feel physically during today's prenatal Pilates session?

Did you notice any changes in your body's flexibility or strength since starting prenatal Pilates?

What thoughts or emotions arose during your prenatal Pilates session?

Space for Creativity
(DOODLES, ILLUSTRATION, TEXT,ETC)

How do you plan to integrate what you've learned in today's session into your daily routine?

How did practicing prenatal Pilates today make you feel about your pregnancy journey?

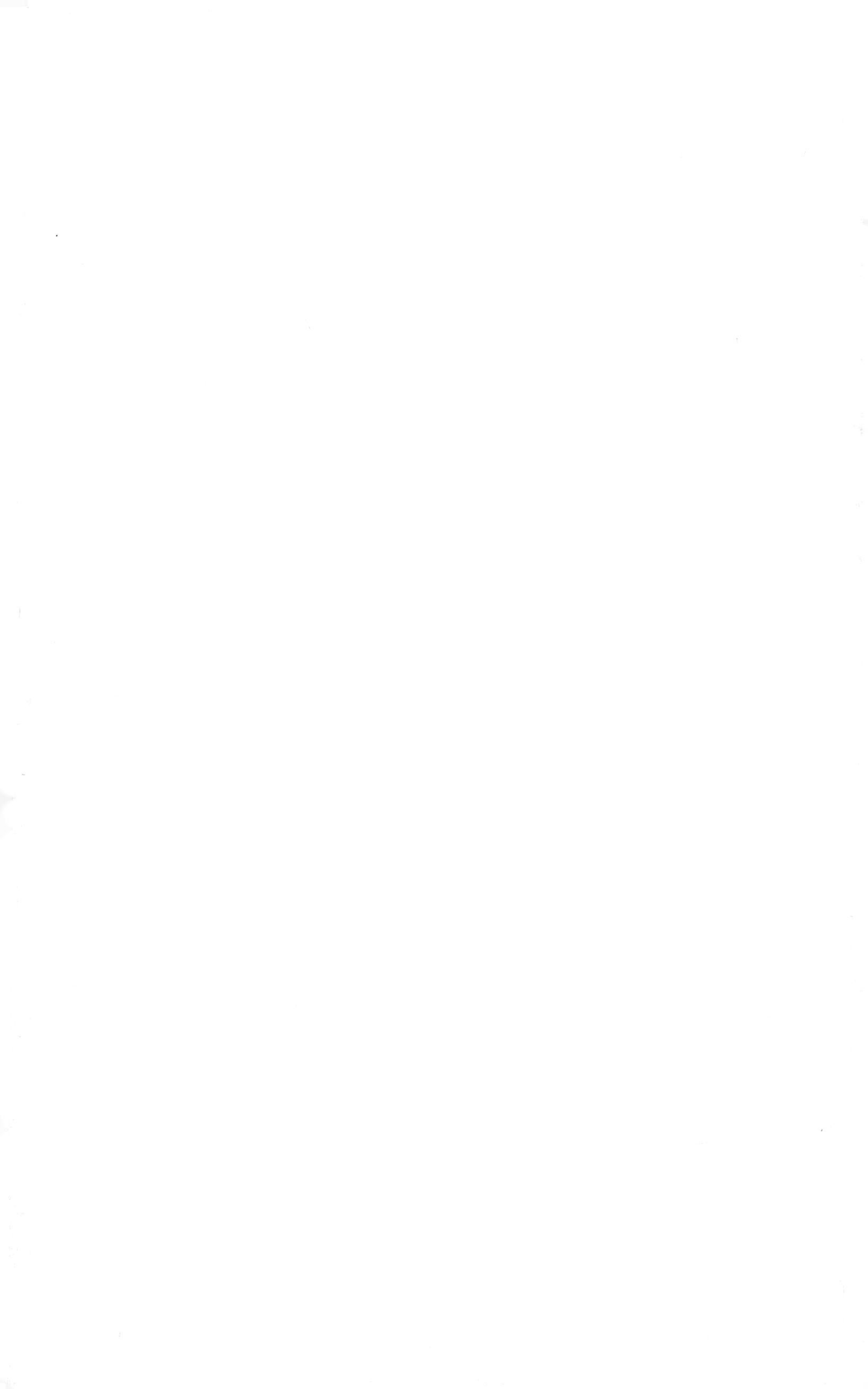

www.ingramcontent.com/pod-product-compliance
Lightning Source LLC
Chambersburg PA
CBHW050819250726
48653CB00006B/2311